BLOOl

AND THEIR TREATMENT,

WITH SPECIAL REFERENCE TO

The Use of Pyrogenium.

BY

J. COMPTON BURNETT, M.D.

"The most summary indication for *Pyrogen* would be to term it the *Aconite* of the typhous or typhoid quality of pyrexia."

JOHN DRYSDALE, M.D.

B. Jain Publishers (P) Ltd.
USA—EUROPE—INDIA

FEVERS AND BLOOD POISONING

7th Impression: 2017

Published by Kuldeep Jain for
B. JAIN PUBLISHERS (P) LTD.
D-157, Sector-63, NOIDA-201307, U.P. (INDIA)
Tel.: +91-120-4933333 • *Email:* info@bjain.com
Website: **www.bjain.com**
Registered office: 1921/10, Chuna Mandi, Pahargani,
New Delhi-110 055 (India)

Printed in India by
J.J. Offset Printers

ISBN: 978-81-319-0786-3

PREFACE.

For several years I have been using *Pyrogenium* in Typhoid Fever and in cases of presumably septic Blood-poisoning; but as my opportunities for observing fevers are few and far between, I had no intention of publishing my observations, believing that some colleagues, who have more to do with Continued Fevers than myself, would soon come forward with the results of large experience with this powerful agent; but I have waited and waited, and on inquiry find that *Pyrogenium* as a therapeutic agent is practically an unknown quantity. As Dr Drysdale, of Liverpool, first introduced *Pyrogenium* to the notice of the profession I looked to the North for information as to its clinical value, but in vain. A while since, my own stock of *Pyrogenium* running short, I caused inquiries to be made in the North with the view of obtaining a fresh supply, but was informed that *Pyrogenium* had not stood the test of experience, was worthless, in fact, and had been given up as therapeutically non-viable. The cause of this adverse judgment I shall not inquire into, merely contenting myself with saying that it will have to be reversed, for I have found that *Pyrogenium* is indeed "the *Aconite* of the typhous or typhoid quality of pyrexia," as Drysdale so tersely puts it.

Experience teaches that over-praise is the bane that blights new remedies, and I would therefore be very chary in praising *Pyrogenium* too much, still I have more than half a conviction that the action of *Pyrogenium* in the pyrexia from blood-poisoning comes very near to one's conception of a specific: however, let it go forth and fight its own battles, which I think it is well able to do.

Hearing that Dr Shuldham, of Putney, had had some practical experience with *Pyrogenium*, I wrote to him to inquire what that might be, and his kind and ready reply will be found at the end of this pamphlet. I shall be glad to insert in any future editions of these pages the experience of any colleagues who may favour me with their results.

Two of the leading homœopathic chemists of London have very kindly prepared the remedy for me, and *Pyrogenium* may therefore be obtained through any homœopathic chemist in the Kingdom, and all the principal ones in the metropolis have it in stock. Those pharmaceutical chemists who may wish to prepare it themselves will find full directions in Dr Drysdale's brochure, but the control experiment on mice should not be omitted, and the dilutions should be made right away, and *not* with glycerine.

I recommend the ordinary sixth centesimal homœopathic dilution, five drops in a dessert-spoonful of water administered every two hours, which is quite harmless, and may be given to the youngest and most delicate baby.

In the following pages I give only as many details as seem to me needful to enable my readers to form an independent judgment as to the value of *Pyrogenium* in pyrexia.

J. COMPTON BURNETT.

REFERENCE TO REMEDIES

Acon. 7, 9, 13, 20, 22, 26, 28, 29, 30, 31, 46.

Actea. 46.

Ars. 9, 13.

Atropin 23.

Bapt. 8, 13, 30. 31, 51.

Bel. 13, 54, 55.

Bry. 46.

Chelid. 28.

Eau-de-Cologne 33, 37.

Gels. 9, 13.

Hydrastis 41.

Merc. 9, 28, 46.

Merc. Biniod 54.

Merc. Iod. 55.

Phos. 9.

Phyto. 30.

Puls. 28.

Pyrogen (pyrexin or Sepsin) 10, 11, 13, 14, 17, 20, 21, 23, 25, 27, 31, 32, 36, 42, 43, 44, 45, 47, 48, 49, 50, 51, 52, 53, 54, 55.

Quinine 13, 20.

Serpent poisons 9.

Vinegar 33, 37.

FEVERS AND BLOOD-POISONING.

H AD the homœopaths done nothing in practical medicine but fix and precisionize the use of *Aconitum* in inflammations and fevers of the inflammatory kind, they would have well merited the undying gratitude of the whole human race. That the use of *Aconite* is thus by them fixed with scientific precision is a matter of common knowledge, and needs no further insisting upon, for "we do not drink our *Aconite* out of a Wilksian mug."

But while this is a fact, while we thus have inflammatory fever, as it were, under our thumbs, we have heretofore had to deal with typhoid and other continued fevers from blood-poisoning in quite a different manner.

Granted that *Aconitum* is no mean remedy even in these continued fevers, still it will not jugulate them or shorten their course, though it *will* ease them, and will even do a good deal towards rendering a mild case milder, perhaps, through the diaphoresis.

Granted also that *Baptisia tinctoria* will do much good in some cases of continued fevers, perhaps even jugulate some gastro-catarrhal cases, still, from a good deal of experience, I can say that it is at best a long way from having a real control over the continued fevers I have met with.

The allopathic treatment of continued fevers is hopeless helplessness: the patients just live or die according to the ratio of the dose of fever-cause to their body-bulk, and (the dose not being of necessity lethal) in proportion to their powers of resistance, and modified by hygienic surroundings. Of course *no* system of therapeutics can be of *any* service where the causal quantity is necessarily fatal right off. "Nursing" is their sheet-anchor!

In modern modish medicine it has come to this state of despair in the treatment of continued fevers. This I have seen in the best hospitals in Europe, and under the best allopathic physicians modern time has produced. I will not deny but that judgment and care, and some clever clinician's resourcefulness, will at times save a given case at a collateral crisis, but this is all that can be truthfully conceded.

Hydropathy does some good in continued fevers, but its help is not very certain.

Homœopathy has hitherto won but few real laurels from its successes in continued fevers, though with the aid of *Baptisia, Arsenicum,* the serpent poisons, *Mercurius, Gelseminum, Aconite, Phosphorus,* and many other more or less symptomatically or hypothetically indicated remedies, the homœopathic practitioners get the best results yet obtained, and bad they are. No one of the remedies used will, even theoretically, cover the whole case. To conduct a case of typhoid to its termination, we often need the aid of a dozen different remedies for the different symptoms and syndromes as they arise, and then the patient will often die at the end, either of diarrhœa and hæmorrhage, or otherwise. And I do not here refer merely to cases amongst the very poor, or under bad or indifferent hygienic surroundings, but to cases in the wealthy classes, with excellent hygienic surroundings, capital nurses, and clever physicians of the most advanced schools of medical thought, and all anxious to do their best.

The fact is, continued fevers are our masters, and we can, even with homœopathy, good nurses, good hygiene, and "the best of everything," only fight the enemy in detail symptomatically or hypothetically. And we thus mitigate the course of the bulk of the cases, and save the lives of a few who, but for our aid, might have succumbed. That homœopathy may be proud even of these achievements I will not deny, but they are not good enough when all put together to make a nice pillow to sleep on. Rather should they fill us with humility and discontent, and stir us all up to find something better.

I was in this frame of mind when Dr Drysdale in and just before the year 1880 brought forward a suggestion that *Pyrexin* might be a good remedy in typhoid and synochus generally. But the dose and mode of administration were stumbling-blocks to me: I did not feel I should like the treatment for my own person, and so I turned away from it not without some feeling of disgust. And, as it is an axiom with me never to give another person a remedy that I would not myself be both willing and anxious to take were I similarly situated, I thought no more of *Pyrexin* as a remedy.

Time passed, and occasional cases of continued fevers—typhoid—came under my sole care or in consultation with other physicians, but I did not cure them, nor could older and more experienced men whom I called to my help. The most experienced and most eminent homœopathic physicians in London kindly saw two consecutive cases very frequently with me; their treatment and mine were practically the same, and also their results— both patients died after a number of weeks of detail treatment that time and again seemed to be curing the cases. But we evidently only cured the symptoms and syndromes—the morbid process was going on within undisturbed in its essential course and progress; the various remedies only acted, as it were, at a tangent, none were adequate, so I made up my mind to go in quest of some better treatment for any future fever cases that might fall to my lot, and Dr Drysdale's *Pyrexin* seemed to stand in the way.

Before going further afield, I thought it best to try the *Pyrexin:* there are strong theoretical grounds for its use in pyrexia quite apart from Dr Drysdale's results, which "have been favourable and give good promise" (p. 16).

Mr Heath, of Ebury Street, very kindly made a preparation of the remedy according to Dr Drysdale's directions ("On Pyrexin or Pyrogen as a Therapeutic Agent," *by John Drysdale, M.D.), and it was carried up to the sixth and twelfth centesimal dilutions and kept ready for my use.

Before I go in to my experience with pyrexin or pyrogen, I think it would be useful to quote from Dr Drysdale's paper; the style is so concise that I cannot advantageously condense the part I want, hence it shall follow in full. Drysdale says,—

"In studying the experimental evidence bearing on the germ theories of disease, I was greatly struck by a remark made by Dr Burdon Sanderson in the *British Medical Journal* of 13th

* London: Bailliere, Tindall, & Cox, 20 King William Street, Strand, W.C., 1880.

February 1875. It was as follows:—'Let me draw your attention to the remarkable fact that no therapeutical agent, no synthetical product of the laboratory, no poison, no drug is known which possesses the property of producing fever. The only liquids which have this endowment are liquids which either contain bacteria, or have a marked proneness to their production.' This last clause is qualified by the statements elsewhere, and from other sources, that the fever-producing agent is a chemical non-living substance formed by living bacteria, but acting independently of any further influence from them, and formed not only by bacteria but also by living pus-corpuscles, or the living blood- or tissue-protoplasm from which these corpuscles spring. This substance when produced by bacteria is the *Sepsin* of Panum and others, but in view of its origin also from pus, and of its fever-producing power, Dr B. Sanderson names it *Pyrogen*. If, however, it is to be also used therapeutically, I suggest the more neutral name of *Pyrexin*. I cannot admit without qualification the statement that no drug of poison can produce fever, for undoubtedly *Aconite, Belladonna, Arsenic, Quinine, Baptisia, Gelseminum,* and a host of other drugs, do produce more or less of the febrile state among other effects. But they produce it only after repeated doses, and contingently on the predisposition of the subject of experiment, and thus uncertainly as regards any individual case or dose; or they produce it as a part of a variety of complex local and general morbid states, of which it may be a secondary phenomenon. It is therefore practically true that no other known substance induces idiopathic pyrexia certainly, directly, and at will after a given dose. This directness and certainty of action ought to make it a remedy of the highest value if it ever can be used therapeutically; and if the law of similars is applicable here as it is in so many other instances, we ought to find it curative in certain states of pyrexia and certain blood-disorders to which its action corresponds pathologically. In order to put this suggestion to the test practically, let us first shortly sum up the symptoms and pathological changes caused by *Sepsin* or *Pyrogen* freed from all bacterial, self-reproductive, or transmissible cause of disease. In a series of experiments by Dr B. Sanderson on dogs after a non-fatal dose of *Pyrogen* (*i.e.* 1¼ cubic centimetre of the aqueous solution per kilogram of body weight, or ½ grain of the solid extract for an ordinary sized dog), the animal shivers and begins to move about restlessly; the temperature rises from 2° to 3° C., the maximum being reached at the end of the third hour. There is great muscular debility; thirst and vomiting come on, followed by feculent and thin mucous, and finally sanguinolent diarrhœa and tenesmus. These symptoms begin to subside in four or five hours, and the animal recovers its normal appetite and liveliness with wonderful rapidity. I mention this fact as proving that the septic poison has not the slightest tendency to multiply in the organism; and, secondly, as rendering it extremely probable that when death occurs it is determined not so much by alvine disorders, which are so prominent, as by the loss of power of the voluntary muscles and of the heart.* Another proof that death when it occurs is from failure of the circulation is, that in non-fatal cases with well-marked gastro-enteric symptoms, the temperature rises gradually during the first four hours, and as gradually subsides; whereas in fatal cases it rises rapidly to 104° F., and then declines rapidly to below the normal before death, thus indicating failure of the heart. In fatal cases from larger doses, the above symptoms increase to intestinal hæmorrhage, purging, collapse, and death. *Post-mortem.*—There is found extravasation of blood in patches underneath the endocardium of the left ventricle, sometimes on the papillary muscles, sometimes

* *Brit. Med. Journ.*, *ii.*, p. 913.

on or in the neighbourhood of the valvular curtains. Similar though less marked appearances are seen in the right ventricle. There are similar points of ecchymosis on the pleura and pericardium. The spleen is enlarged and full of blood. The mucous membrane of the stomach and small intestine is intensely injected with detachment of the epithelium, and exudation of sanguinolent fluid distends the lumen of the gut. These appearances indicate a general tendency to congestion and capillary hæmorrhage as well as locally, congestion and capillary stasis of the gastro-intestinal mucous membrane, with shedding of the epithelium, as the nature of the disorder. The state of the blood plays a great part in the morbid process; it is darker in hue, and the corpuscles arrange themselves in clumps instead of rolls; many of the blood-corpuscles are partially dissolved in the *liquor sanguinis*, communicating to it a red colour: a large quantity of the hæmoglobin is lost by evacuation of the bowels, and conversion into bilirubin; the partial disintegration of the white corpuscles, by liberating the fibrino-plastic ferment, is supposed to be one cause of the capillary stasis.

"The symptomatic and pathological effects are substantially the same in man, and, indeed, the analogy between the symptoms and morbid appearance and state of the blood in septicæmia after wounds and the experimental poisoning with *Sepsin* is very close.

"Now, granting that the powerful agent producing these remarkable effects may be expected to act therapeutically as an alternative in morbid states which present the pathological *simile* to them, what are these morbid states, and how are they to be recognised in the complex phenomena of fever in the human subject? To answer this we must inquire what is the cardinal point in the proximate cause of pyrexia with which we have to deal in employing a directly acting remedy? To this question—at least as regards the chief phenomenon which determines the name pyrexia, viz., the increased heat—the critical review of the experiments of Senator, Leyden, and others by B. Sanderson,* gives a reply.

"The temperature of the body being dependent on the production and discharge of heat. of which the former is a function of living protoplasm, the latter a function of the organs of circulation, respiration, and secretion, the question arises, whether pyrexial increa e of temperature depends upon the former or the latter. To this Dr. B. Sanderson thus replies (p. 45) :—

* See *Blue Book*, 1876, No. 1, Appendix.

'Two possibilities are open to us. One is, that fever originates in disorder of the nervous centres, that by means of the influence of the nervous system on the systemic functions, the liberation of heat at the surface of the body is controlled or restrained, so that "by retention" the temperature rises, and, finally, that the increased temperature so produced acts on the living substance of the body, so as to disorder its nutrition. The other alternative is that fever originates in the living tissues, that it is from first to last a disorder of the protoplasm, and that all the systemic disturbances are secondary. The facts and considerations we have had before us are, I think, sufficient to justify the definitive rejection of the first hypothesis in all its forms; for, on the one hand, we have seen that no disorder of the systemic functions, or of the nervous centres which preside over them, is capable of inducing a state which can be identified with febrile pyrexia; and, on the other, that it is possible for such a state to originate and persist in the organism after the influence of the central nervous system has been withdrawn from the tissues by the severance of the spinal cord. We are, therefore, at liberty to adopt the tissue-origin of fever as the basis on which we hope eventually to construct an explanation of the process.' It is elsewhere concluded that it is in the protoplasm of the blood and the muscles that take place those changes of activity and disintegration on which depend the changes of temperature, and no doubt the other essential phenomena which characterize fever.

"What, therefore, on these data are we to expect from an agent which shall act directly as curative of the pyrexial state? Not certainly any palpable disturbance of the nervous system which can in health lower temperature by promoting heat discharge, as is expected from large doses of *Quinine,* or from the merely physical action of cold baths; nor a general support of the vital powers till the specific disease runs its course, as is expected from alcohol, etc. But, on the contrary, a simple modification of the exalted and perverted protoplasmic action in which the proximate cause of pyrexia consists, which shall be of such a nature as to bring it back to health. Let us assume (without any attempt to prove it, but merely to give an intelligible illustration in explanation) the hypothesis of Beale, that the essence of inflammation and fever consists in a degeneration in the scale of biological development of the bioplasts of the blood and tissues, which involves the production of a more rapidly growing and disintegrating kind of protoplasm; our most complete and perfect conception of a direct remedy would be that of an agent which would act as a specific stimulus to the affected protoplasm, and bring back its germinal development up to the normal plane. This has long been my view of the action of *Aconite* in inflammatory fever, or, at least, that it acted directly on the pyrexically affected protoplasm, and not on the vaso-motor nerves or centres of the heart, or of the spinal marrow; for reiterated experience has shown that it acts in far too small a dose to exert any directly depressant effect on the heart or its nerves, or, indeed, and perceptible effect on them at all. Now, the living matter or protoplasm is capable of an almost infinite variety of kinds of morbid action according to the predisposing and exciting causes acting on it, and hence pyrexia may vary indefinitely in its character, even independently of the addition of the local lesion proper to the concrete specific fevers; so no directly curative remedy can be applicable to more than a few forms, or even to only one, *e.g.*, *Aconite* suits inflammatory fevers, and *Quinine* malarious intermittents, while they would be powerless if interchanged. To what form, then, should we except *Pyrexin* or *Pyrogen* to be applicable? The true clue to this is given, I think, by the state of the blood, for that is the most marked and important of the signs of septicæmia; the local congestions and extravasations not being so constant or so grave as respects the issue. If we contrast the characteristic hyperinotic state of the blood in inflammatory fever, displaying its bright colour, buffy coat, firm coagulum, and the adherence of the red corpuscles in rolls, with the septicæmic state of blood already described, showing its dark and dissolved state, loose coagulum, the red corpuscles adhering in clumps, and the increase of white corpuscles, we shall see well-marked grounds of distinction This latter state of the blood is very similar to, if not identical with, that which belongs to typhous or adynamic fevers, and, indeed, in describing fatal cases of septicæmia after wounds the analogy of the symptoms is so great with these fevers that the word 'typhous' is generally used in describing them. Hence the shortest discrimination of the indications for the use of *Pyrexin* or *Pyrogen* may be stated to be the typhous or typhoid character or quality of pyrexia, using these adjectives in their old-fashioned sense. For although the clinical discrimination of enteric fever from typhus is a great gain, it is unfortunate that the word 'typhoid' should have been appropriated to the former, as it either introduces confusion into our nomenclature or deprives us of a hitherto well-understood expression of the character of pyrexia as distinct from the name of a specific disease. We shall find it convenient to go back to the terms of Cullen, viz., synocha for inflammatory fever, the typhous or typhoid condition for the low adynamic or asthenic character or quality of fever, and synochus for the mixed kind, which is inflammatory at the beginning and typhous at the end. I do not know that the more accurate discrimination of the typhous, enteric, and relapsing fevers into distinct specific diseases gives any ground for denying the existence of the above distinctions of character in the pyrexial state in general, and, therefore, we should still keep up the words inflammatory and typhous or typhoid, as expressive of different qualities or characters of fever, and not of distinct febrile diseases.

"As *Aconite* is well known to be the most important of the remedies for the synochal or inflammatory pyrexia, so the most summary indication for *Pyrogen* would be to term it the *Aconite* of the typhous or typhoid quality of pyrexia. This being a condition and not a distinct disease, it is to be looked for as occurring in a variety of diseases such as the typhous and enteric fevers themselves always, and more or less it may occur in intermittents, so-called bilious remittents, in certain varieties or stages of the exanthemata, especially scarlatina, measles, and smallpox, of dysentery, and of epidemic

pneumonias, diphtheria, etc. From the gastro-
enteric symptoms *Pyrogen* may possibly also
apply to some stage of cholera and to yellow
fever. It is, of course, to be distinctly under-
stood that this substance is only recommended.
at certain stages and phases of these diseases,
and entirely as a remedy of a secondary or
subordinate character, and not in any sense as a
specific for the whole disease.

"*Sepsin* or *Pyrogen*, it must be remembered,
is only a chemical poison, like *Atropin* or serpent
venom, whose action is definite and limited by
the dose, and it is incapable of inducing an indefinitely reproducible disease in minimal dose,
after the manner of the special poisons of the
specific fevers; its sphere, therefore, is by no
means commensurate with that of these diseases,
and if ever true specifics for them should be dis-
covered, it is hardly probable that such would be
merely chemical non-living agents. At present
there is no question at all of such specifics. The
only point is that we should be able to form an
intelligible idea of the way in which a margin
can be supposed to exist in individual cases, say
of enteric fever, smallpox, or yellow fever, etc.,
in which a directly acting medicine can do good
to the pyrexia without at the same time having
any power to check, modify, or shorten the true
specific disease. Observation, I think, shows

that such a margin exists, for we are all familiar with the immense variety in the degree of severity, especially as regards the pyrexia existing between cases of the same specific fever in different individuals, while at the same time the cardinal symptoms are pronounced sufficiently to leave no doubt of the diagnosis, and the completeness of the specific process is also shown by the protection against subsequent attacks being as complete after the slight cases as after the more severe. In scarlatina and smallpox both these circumstances are notorious, and the astonishing mildness of the pyrexia in some cases of enteric fever, in which the local diseased process runs its full course, is well known.

"When we take these facts in connexion with the theory of Beale that not all—nay, not even the majority—of the new bioplasts, whose formation and continued multiplication constitutes the essence of fever and inflammation, are, in a specific contagious disease, themselves specific, and capable of conveying the disease, we can easily see that there may be in each specific fever a large margin of non-specific febrile action or protoplasmic change. It may be, and probably is, this which gives the severity and fatality to certain cases by its excessive amount rather than the greater intensity of the specific process, owing to increased susceptibilities of the patient towards the specific poison, although no doubt that is also a factor of importance in the variations of severity in different individuals. At all events, we easily see from the above considerations the reasonableness of the expectation that any remedy which could moderate and control the concomitant non-specific pyrexia in the specific fevers would thereby palpably diminish the average mortality, even though it could not cut short the specific disease itself. Whether *Pyrogen* be such a remedy remains to be seen; at present we have only to show that a place is open for a possible agent of this kind. Our expectations, also, must not be pitched too high, because, for innumerable reasons, as we all know, a considerable mortality must attend all the severe specific fevers, and the margin wherein positive curative treatment adds to the value of good negative treatment is not large. Besides, from the very character of the symptoms and stage of the disease for which this remedy is indicated, it must often be in the position of a forlorn hope. Therefore it is only by the statistical comparison of a large number of cases that we can determine how far lives have been saved by it.

"The known specific fevers do not by any means exhaust the possible sphere of a remedy for the 'typhous' condition of pyrexia; for, although it is no longer the fashion to speak of the synochus of Cullen, yet, as far as my experience goes (and I doubt not other practitioners will agree with me), the list of species or varieties of continued fever in this country is by no means exhausted when we name the inflammatory, rheumatic, typhus, enteric, and relapsing. On the contrary, we all meet with cases of fever which cannot be distinctly referred to local lesion, and cannot be fairly brought under any of the above names, and for want of a more definite appellation we have to speak of as catarrhal, gastric, or bilious fever, or describe in some such vague way. Many of these are synochal, and require *Aconite* at the outset, while in the later stages a more adynamic state sets in, supposed to require stimulants, thus corresponding to the synochus of Cullen. In the specific fevers also, there may occur more or less of this primary and secondary quality of the pyrexia requiring *Aconite* at the first stage and (should our anticipation prove correct) *Pyrogen* at the later stages. Doubtless Cullen, his contemporaries, and for long his successors, described and treated as synochus many cases of continued fever, which were, in reality, enteric, or even relapsing, before Henderson separated the latter or Jenner the former, from the general mass of continued fevers; and, no doubt, we are all doing the same in respect to other species to be discriminated in future. But this is of less consequence as regards medicinal treatment as long as we are guided by indications for a particular quality of pyrexia, and not the concrete disease in which that may occur. If the discrimination of enteric fever as a species may be correctly held to explain away synochus in part, yet can we admit that the supervention of bacterial growth at the later stage will account for all the rest? Certainly, in that case, the sepsin of the bacteria would produce a state of blood analogous to the 'typhous' state, and if itself the cause would of course exclude our remedy."

I make no apology for appropriating so much of Dr Drysdale's little treatise "On Pyrexin or Pyrogen as a Therapeutic Agent." as I should not like either to hold its author responsible for my views as to the value in pyrexia of this new and powerful agent, or to appear to claim his.

Let us now go to what evidence I myself have of the *clinical value of Pyrogen*.

Miss C. M. A., æt. twelve years and eleven months, was taken ill in *February* 1885 at her parents' seat in Sussex—one of the healthiest spots in the country. On the night of *Monday the 16th* she had a headache; felt hot and sick, and could not sleep.

On Tuesday the 17th she went to London for the day; felt sick, cold, and hysterical on her homeward journey; was very sick on reaching home; had headache; was restless, and talked a good deal in her sleep. Her mother gave her *Pulsatilla.*

On Wednesday the 18th she stayed in bed to breakfast; she was feverish, disinclined for food, and hysterical; complained of pain in her abdomen; all her bones ached; her legs felt as if she could not move them. Her mother gave her *Aconite* and *Chelidonium* in alternation.

On Thursday the 19th she was much the same as on the preceding day; she cried a good deal; fancied she saw mice and people about in her bedroom; tongue thickly coated; cannot bear any talking, noise, or light. Her mother continued with the *Aconite,* but substituted *Merc. sol.* for the *Chelidonium.*

On Friday the 20th I find this note recorded: Did not sleep last night for more than half an hour at a time; muttered and talked and tossed about in her sleep; complains of headache; pains in her back, arms, and jaws; she dozes for a few minutes and then awakes wandering in her mind; will partake of nothing but water and a little milk.

P.M.
6   T. 103·2°
8.45 T. 104°
11   T. 103·4°

With an *Aconite-resisting* temperature of 103° to 104° the child's mother—a clever, capable, and altogether a remarkable woman—knew that danger was ahead. She knew well, from practical life-experience, that when *Aconite* fails to bring down the fever, you must prepare for the enemy of pyrexia properly so-called, or for a more or less serious something. Accordingly the local allopathic medical man was called in, and he very carefully examined the patient, but found nothing but a spot on the left tonsil. The temperature he found to be 103·4° and the pulse 132. In the absence of pain or distinct feature beyond the pyrexia, he gave as his opinion that it was an attack of herpes, of which he had had some cases in the neighbourhood, and in which the fever ran rapidly up as high as he found Miss A's., and then became normal as rapidly as it had run up, and he expressed, accordingly, the hope that this case would do the same.

The patient having had *Aconite* for five days, she was put upon *Baptisia* and *Phytolacca* on Friday evening. Patient's tongue was very foul, coated in the centre, strawberry-like round the edges; breath offensive; had aching.

On Saturday the 21*st* the *Baptisia* and the *Phyto*. were continued till I arrived and took charge of the case at 6.15 P.M., and a sister from Mildmay took night duty from this date on.

The record of temperature on Saturday 21st is this—

A.M.
10   T. 104°
12   T. 103·2°

P.M.
2   T. 103·6°
5   T. 104·4°
8   T. 104·4°

After going over the already given history of the case and its course, and seeing that *Aconite* and *Baptisia* had done no good, and after a due examination of the patient, it was very clear that we had to do with a case of gastric fever of the gravest kind.

Had Rademacher or Kissel, Guttceit or Rapp been living and practising in the neighbourhood, I think it likely, highly probable, that they would have known the right remedy corresponding to the epidemic genius of the disease. But I had no means of knowing what that genius was, or its corresponding remedy; and with a nearly constant temperature rising to almost 105 degrees Fahrenheit, there was no time to be lost, the less so as the temperature had been slowly and steadily rising for days.

Beginning at 9 P.M. on Saturday the 21st, five drops of *Pyrogenium* 6 was given every two hours.

Diet ordered was: beef-tea, chicken-tea, water, juice of apples, and grapes. Also cold water compress to abdomen, to be renewed every four hours.

In view of the very great importance of the question under consideration, viz., the efficacy or non-efficacy of this power-ful agent in true typhoid—in the treat-ment of which all therapeutists to date have had to sing so small—I propose to give the day-book kept at the time in the sick-room verbatim.

Sunday, 22nd.

1	A.M.	Medicine (*Pyrogen* 6).
2	,,	T. 104°.
		Slept.
4	,,	Medicine.
6	,,	Medicine.
8	,,	T. 103·6°; beef-tea, 1½ oz.
8.40	,,	Medicine.
10.40	,,	Medicine.
11.10	,,	Apple water.
12		T. 104·4°; beef-tea.
12.40	P.M.	Medicine.
1.25	,,	T. 104°; sponged; apple water.
1.50	,,	Chicken-tea, 1½ oz.
2.35	,,	Medicine; compress.
3	,,	Passed water.
		Slept ¼ hour; delirious.
3.50	,,	Beef-tea, 1½ oz.
4.35	P.M.	T. 104·4°; medicine.
5.45	,,	Chicken-tea.
6.30	,,	Medicine.
8.30	,,	T. 103·4°.

9.15 P.M. Chicken-tea; compress.

9.45 „ T. 104°.

10 „ Medicine.

11 „ Apple water.

Very restless, wishing to get out of bed.

12 „ Medicine.

Asks to have her mouth wiped out with vinegar and water constantly, "it feels so slimy." Head aching. Has rags constantly on forehead and face sponged with Eau-de-Cologne and water. At her request washed her feet.

Monday, 23rd.

1.30 A.M. Chicken-tea; passed water.

2 „ Medicine; less restless. Slept ½ hour

4.15 „ Medicine.

4.45 „ Chicken-tea, 2 oz.

6.15 „ Medicine; passed water.

8 „ T. 101°.

8.10 „ Medicine.

9.40 „ Beef-tea and Murdock's food, 2 oz.

10.30 „ Medicine.

12 T. 102·4°; chicken-tea, 2 oz.

12.40 P.M. Medicine.

2.15 „ Beef-tea and Murdock, 1½ oz.

2.35 „ T. 103°.

2.55 P.M. Medicine; passed water.
4   ,,   T. 103°.
4.20 ,,   Chicken-tea, 2 oz.
4.55 ,,   Medicine.
5.30 ,,   Passed water.
6.25 ,,   Beef-tea and Murdock, 3 oz.
7.15 ,,   Medicine.
8   ,,   T. 101·6°.
           Slept 20 minutes.
9.30 ,,   Medicine.
10   ,,   Chicken-tea, 2 oz.
11.30 ,,   Medicine.
12   ,,   T. 100·8°.
           Passed a good deal of water; char-
               acter changed; very high colour,
               but less thick on standing.

Tuesday, 24th.

1.45 A.M. Medicine; passed water.
           Slept ½ hour.
2.15 ,,   Slept 20 minutes.
3.15 ,,   Chicken-tea; slept 45 minutes.
4   ,,   Medicine.
           Slept 45 minutes.
6   ,,   Medicine; passed water.
6.30 ,,   Chicken-tea.
8   ,,   T. 98·2°.
8.10 ,,   Beef-tea, 2 oz.
9   ,,   Medicine.

10.15 A.M. Beef-tea and Murdock, 3 oz.

12   T. 100°.

12.15 P.M. Medicine.

1   ,,   Chicken-tea, 2 oz.

2   ,,   T. 101°·

      Slept.

3.30 ,, Medicine; passed water.

4   ,,   T. 102·4°.

4.10 ,, Beef-tea and Murdock, 3 oz.

6.30 ,, T. 100·8°.

7   ,,   Chicken-tea, 2 oz.

7.30 ,, Medicine.

8   ,,   T. 100°·

9.15 ,, Beef-tea and Murdock, 2 oz.

11.10 ,, Medicine.

      Slight action of bowels, full of bile.
         Passed water.

      Medicine to be taken every 4 hours
         instead of every 2 hours. Says
         she has no headache now.

Wednesday, 25th.

1   A.M. Chicken-tea, 2 oz.; slept 1¼ hours.

3.25 ,, Medicine; slept 2 hours.

4   ,,   Chicken-tea, 2 oz.

      Slept an hour and a half.

7.20 ,, Medicine.

7.45 ,, Beef-tea and Murdock, 2 oz.

8   ,,   T. 99·8°.

10.45 A.M. Chicken-tea, 2 oz.

11.15 „ Medicine.

12 T. 99·6°.

1 P.M. Beef-tea and Murdock, 3 oz.

1.15 „ T. 98·6°; passed water.

3.15 „ Medicine.

3.45 „ Chicken-tea, 2 oz. Very thirsty.

4 „ T. 100·8°.

5 „ T. 101°.

6.15 „ Beef-tea and Murdock, 3 oz; passed water.

7 „ Medicine (*New Pyrogenium,* No. 12).

8 „ T. 100·8°.

Slept off and on.

10.55 „ Medicine.

11.30 „ Chicken-tea, 2 oz.

12 „ T. 99·4°.

Pyrogenium, No. 12, to be given every three hours in five-drop doses. Asks constantly for claret cup. A juicy plum. Drank a great deal of water, lemon water, and apple water.

Thursday, 26th.

2 A.M. Medicine. Slept.

4 „ Chicken-tea, 2 oz.; passed water.

5 „ Medicine.

6 „ Chicken-tea, 2 oz.

6.50 A.M. T. 99˙4°.

8.20 ,, Medicine.

8.20 ,, T. 97˙2°.

8.50 ,, Beef-tea and Murdock, 3 oz.

9 ,, T. 98˙2°.

10.50 ,, Chicken-tea, 2 oz.

11.20 ,, Medicine.

Asleep ½ hour.

12.30 P.M. T. 99˙4°.

12.50 ,, Beef-tea and Murdock, 3 oz.

2.25 ,, Medicine; passed water.

2.50 ,, Chicken-tea, 2 oz.

4 ,, T. 101°; little chicken and rice.

5.25 ,, Medicine.

6 ,, Beef-tea and Murdock, 2 oz.; bread and butter.

8 ,, T. 100°; chicken-tea, 2 oz.

8.50 ,, Medicine.

Slept 2½ hours.

12 ,, Medicine.

Craving for bread and butter. Has ceased to use the Eau-de-Cologne and rags to her forehead, and sponging face and hands—hitherto she used them constantly. A smaller quantity of water passed.

Friday, 27th.

12.30 A.M. Chicken-tea, 2 oz.

Slept 2 hours and 1½ hours.

5   A.M. Medicine.
5.30 „   Chicken-tea, 2 oz.
7.15 „   T. 98°.
8.10 „   Medicine; passed water.
8.30 „   T. 97·4°.
8.45 „   Beef-tea and Murdock; bread and
          butter.
10.15 „   T. 97·4°.
11   „   Brandy, raw egg, and milk in all, 2 oz.
11.30 „   Medicine.
12   T. 99·8°.
1   P.M. T. 99·4; chicken-tea, 2 oz.; bread
          and butter. Slept.
3.15 „   Beef-tea and Murdock.
4   „   T. 100·4°; passed water.
5   „   T. 100·4°.
6   „   Chicken-tea, 2 oz.
7   „   Medicine and compress.
7.40 „   Beef-tea and Murdock.
8   „   T. 99·8.
11.15 „   Medicine.
          Telegram from Dr Burnett to take
              off compress and discontinue
              medicine till he arrives at 6.15 P.M.
              No thirst to-day, has not once
              asked for a drink.

Saturday, 28th.

12.5 A.M. Chicken-tea, 2 oz.
          Slept 4 hours.

4.35 A.M. Medicine.

5.5 „ Chicken-tea, 2 oz.

7.30 „ Medicine.

7.50 „ T. 98·4°; compress.

8 „ Beef-tea and Murdock, 3 oz.; bread and butter.

8.15 „ T. 97·4°.

10.30 „ T. 97·4°; medicine; passed water.

11.30 „ Beef-tea and Murdock; bread and butter, 3 oz.

12 T. 97·2°.

1.30 P.M. Medicine.

1.45 „ T. 97·8°.

2 „ Brandy, raw egg, and milk, 1½ oz.

3.30 „ Chicken-tea, 2 oz.

4 „ T. 98·4°.

5 „ T. 98·6°; grapes; bread and butter.

5.30 „ Passed water.

5.40 „ Beef-tea, Murdock, bread and butter, 3 oz.

6.30 „ T. 99°; medicine; compress.

8.30 „ T. 98·4°; chicken-tea, 2 oz.

Sunday, March 1st.

12.30 A.M. Chicken-tea, 2 oz.

3.10 „ Chicken-tea, 2 oz.

6.45 „ Chicken-tea, 2 oz.

8 „ T. 97·2°.

8-15 „ Egg, brandy, and bread and butter, 1½ oz.

9.30 A.M. T. 96·6°.

10.10 „ Beef-tea, Murdock 4 oz.; bread and water; passed water.

11   „ T. 96·8°.

12   T. 96·8°; chicken-tea, 2 oz.; chicken sandwich; water, 2 oz.

1.30 P.M. T. 97°; came out in a rash on the left arm from the shoulder to the wrist.

2   „ Beef-tea and Murdock, 4 oz.; bread and butter; water, 2 oz.

4   „ T. 97·6°; chicken-tea, 2 oz.; chicken sandwich; water, 2 oz.

5   „ T. 98°.

6   „ An apple.

6.45 „ T. 97·8°; beef-tea and Murdock, 4 oz.; bread and butter; water, 2 oz.

7   „ Passed water, natural in colour.

7.30 „ T. 97·6°; egg, brandy, and milk, 2 oz.
      Sunday.—Slept all last night; gave chicken-tea twice without rousing her. Urine high coloured and quantity much less. Urine passed at 7 o'clock, a pale natural colour. Asked if she might get up to-morrow as she feels quite well. Passed 20 oz. urine.

Monday March 2nd.

12.15 A.M. Has slept since 8 o'clock.

1   „ Beef-tea, 2 oz.

6   A.M. Beef-tea, 2 oz.
7   ,,   T. 96·4°.
7.10 ,,   Egg, brandy, and milk, 2 oz.
8   ,,   T. 97·2°.
9.10 ,,   Beef-tea and Murdock, 4 oz.; bread
           and butter.
10   ,,   T. 96·6°; passed water.
11.30 ,,   Chicken-tea, 4 oz.; bread and butter.
12   T. 97°.
           Slept 2½ hours.
3   P.M. T. 97·4°; beef-tea and Murdock, 4 oz.;
           bread and butter.
3.30 ,,   Medicine, Hydrastis φ 2 drops.
4   ,,   T. 97·2°.
5.30 ,,   Chicken-tea, 4 oz; chicken sandwiches.
6   ,,   T. 97°; medicine.
7   ,,   T. 97·4°.
7.30 ,,   Egg, brandy, and milk, 2 oz.
8   ,,   T. 96·2°; medicine passed water.
           Began Hydrastis φ 2 drop doses.
           Urine clear. At 8 o'clock com-
           plained of being very tired, and
           asked to go back to her bed.

Tuesday, 3rd.

1   A.M. Chicken-tea, 2 oz.
5   ,,   Chicken-tea, 2 oz.
7   ,,   Medicine.
8   ,,   Beef-tea and Murdock, 4 oz.; bread
           and butter and apple.

8   A.M. T. 97·4°.
- 9.30 ,, Medicine.
10   ,, Egg, brandy, and milk, 2 oz; bread
            and butter.
11.30 ,, Medicine.
12   T. 98·2°.
12.15 P.M. Chicken-tea, 4 oz., and sandwish.
1.30 ,, Medicine.
2   ,, T. 98·2°.
            Asleep for ½ hour.
3.15 ,, Beef-tea and Murdock, 4 oz.
3.45 ,, Medicine.

I will now tabulate the temperature-
markings, not in the form of a curve, but
in figures according to days:—

o'Clock.	Fri.	Sat.	Sun.	Mon.	Tues	Wed.
A.M.						
8.	..	104°	103·6°	101°	98·2°	99·8°
12.	..	103·2°	104·4°	102·4°	100°	99·6°
P.M.						
4.	..	103·6°	104·4°	103°	102·4°	100·8°
8.	104°	104·4°	104°	101·6°	100°	100·8

	Thurs.	Fri.	Sat.	Sun.	Mon.
A.M.					
8.	98·2°	97·4°	97·4°	97·2°	97·2°
12.	99·4°	99·8°	97·2°	96·8°	97°
P.M.					
4.	101°	100·4°	98·4°	97·6°	97·2°
8.	100°	99·8°	98·4°	97·6°	96·2°

REMARKS.—The febrifuge and otherwise the curative action of the *Pyrogen*
was soon manifest, and the normal

temperature was reached within a week, and then came the subnormal reaction. Whether others will believe that *Pyrogen* here acted curatively I do not know. I personally am satisfied that the remedy broke up the fever, and, humanly speaking, saved the young lady's life. That is also the opinion of the mother, who has large experience.

But the nurses were experienced in fever also, and they should be able to judge to some extent. In order to know the nurses' opinions, I wrote to the young lady's mother for information on the subject, and this is the reply,—

"Feb. 2, 1888.

"The Mildmay nurses could not make it out; they felt sure —— had typhoid for one reason and then another, and that it must last such a time; then, when *Pyrogen* did for the course they considered it absolutely necessary for typhoid to take, they were shut up to the correction that after all it was only a good imitation, and not the genuine fever!"

However, let us pass on to some further clinical work done by *Pyrogen:* one case counts but for very little, it is so easy to be mistaken or be deceived, and *experientia fallax* is a very hoary saw.

CASE II.—Subsequently a middle-aged gentleman had an attack of fever, but it was complicated with, or arising from an enlarged liver with old peritonitic adhesions and adhesions of Glisson's capsule. In this case the hepatic and other remedies of a more constitutional action did not seem to act, and so I fell back upon *Pyrogen,* with the result that the other remedies then acted well, and patient made a quick recovery. Looking now back on this case, I am disposed to think that it was a mild septic fever supervening upon chronic hypertrophy of the liver, and the liver was not able to right itself till the continued fever had been quelled by the *Pyrogen.* This case I will not dwell upon, as the evidence it affords does not count for much.

CASE III.—This case, K. W. A., occurred subsequently in the same house as Case I., and the patient was at the time about 13 years of age, and he is brother of the subject mentioned in Case I.

I will also not dwell long on K. W. A.'s case, or give any particulars further than to say, that the giving of *Pyrogen* was followed at once by a distinct drop in the temperature of nearly three degrees, and it did not again go up, but remained at about 99.0° for many weeks, when the patient got well, and is now a strong fellow.

For the sake of making the case comprehensible, I will just add that from the course of the case, from the remedies that helped, and from those that did not, I am of opinion that patient had continued fever which started mesenteric mischief, and that the pyrexia 102.6° was cured by *Pyrogen;* whereas the slight febrile movement that went on for so many weeks— nearly nine—was consequent upon chronic inflammation in the mesenteric glands. There was much obstinate diarrhœa. However, whatever the nature of the case was, the exhibition of *Pyrogen* was followed by a drop of three degrees in the temperature.

Still I would not attach much importance to this case either.

CASE IV.—William R. A., æt. 19, oddly enough also of the same family as the foregoing, but residing at, Kensington. He came home (to Kensington) early from office, complaining of neuralgia, on the afternoon of Wednesday, the 17th February 1886. Did not sleep that night, and so did not get up to breakfast next morning, when his temperature was found to be 100˙6°.

As he seemed to have a feverish cold, complained of pains in his bones, he was ordered *Aconite* and *Bryonia*. Temperature at 5 P.M. 101°, when Dr ——— was sent for, and patient was got up stairs: he had been sleeping in the smoking room adjoining the W.C. since February 2nd. The doctor ordered *Actaea* and *Bryonia*. Did not sleep much on Thursday night.

Friday.—The doctor saw him in the morning, and changed the medicines to *Merc. viv.* 3x trit., as much as would lie on a sixpence, every four hours. On *Saturday, Aconite* was alternated with it every hour. Slept indifferently.

On *Sunday,* patient, was removed to higher ground, viz., close to Cavendish

Square. Patient bore the removal well, but profuse perspirations broke out from time to time, great aching in his limbs, headache from time to time all over forehead, great thirst, breath foul, tongue not much coated but brownish, gets depressed if left alone, and breaks out in perspiration; pain in the stomach at times, bowels rumble a great deal, nose bleeds readily, throat sore and congested, gum ragged where wisdom tooth has lately come through, gets a pain if he drinks cold milk, jaws very stiff, so much so that he cannot separate his teeth but a very little.

The physician in charge was very positive that it was a case of true typhoid, and I may say that the gentleman in question has had special experience of typhoid, and knows it better than many physicians. There was a regular staff of hospital nurses in attendance experienced in fevers, and they were quite sure it was real typhoid.

The young man's mother having seen the effects of *Pyrogen* in continued fevers —the cases I have already related—told the physician in charge about it, and wanted him to give *Pyrogen,* but he refused, saying that it was quite impossible to stop typhoid fever, and that, therefore, this case would have to run its course. But the lady was so sure that she had seen *Pyrogen* break up fever, that she did not feel it would be right to go on without at least trying it, and the doctor thereupon withdrew from the case. And as I had long been the ordinary medical adviser of the family, and being, moreover, the foster parent of *Pyrogen*, I was asked to take up the case, which I was sorry to do on the one hand, but rather keen to try my friend *Pyrogen* again all the same. This was Monday morning, February 22, 1886. Up to this date the temperature-markings were:—

o'Clock.	18th.	19th.	20th.	21st.	22nd.
A.M.					
8.	100·6°	100·2°	100·8°	100·1°	100·4°
12.	100·8°	100·6°	100·1°	100·1°	100°
P.M.					
4.	101°	100·4°	101°	100·6°	
8.	100·8°	100·2°	101°	100·6°	

At two o'clock on the afternoon of 22nd *Pyrogen* was begun, five drops of No. 6 in water every two hours, and I saw the patient in the afternoon for the first time. The very pose of the patient, his mode of lying in bed, spoke clearly in favour of his complaint being typhoid: he lay on his back in listless indifference as if his body were not his, and it were sinking almost through the bed. The temperature went down already in a few hours, becoming practically normal in three days, and patient slept for three hours after the sixth dose. Here is the complete record of the temperature,—

o'Clock	18th.	19th.	20th.	21st.	22nd.	23rd.	24th.
A.M.							
8.	100·6°	100·2°	100·8°	101°	100·4°	..	99·4° 98·8°
12.	100·8°	100·6°	101°	101°	100°	99·6°	99° 99·4°
P.M.							
4.	101°	100·4°	101°	100·6°	100°	100·2°	99·4° 99·2°
8.	100·8°	100·2°	101°	100·6°	100°	99·6°	98·8°

o'Clock	25th.	26th.	27th.	28th.	March 1st.	2nd.	
A.M.							
8.	98·2°	98°	97·8°	98·2°	97·4°	97·6°	98·6°
12.	98·6°	97·8°	98·6°	98°	97·4°	97·4°	98·6°
P.M.							
4.	98·8°	98·6°	98·4°	98·4°	97·4°	97·2°	97·4°
8.	..	98·4°	..	..	98·4°	97·2°	97·6°

I *do* attach *very* great importance to this case, as it was most manifest that the *Pyrogen* acted curatively even though we had taken no notice of the temperature at all; the patient soon got sleep, picked up, took an interest in his surroundings, wanted food; kidneys and bowels and skin all told that the fever was not being treated merely by it, but jugulated, snuffed out, if I may so say.

No doubt I may be inclined to think too much of it, but my duty is done when I give my evidence and my opinion.

I had to wait some time after this before suitable cases of fever presented themselves for a further and more extended trial of *Pyrogen,* and I felt somewhat disappointed at not seeing any clinical results obtained by it brought to the notice of the profession either by Dr Drysdale himself or by other colleagues. So I determined to wait till such were forthcoming, but I waited in vain, nothing came. However, *tout vient a celui qui sait attendre,* and in December 1887 I had the good fortune to be called in to treat two young ladies in London both with continued fever, the temperature in one case being 104° to 105°, and in the other ranging from 99° to 101.°

CASES V. and VI.—The young ladies had been under allopathic treatment, and the fever would not lessen. Having them both in adjoining rooms, and both cases being clearly of common origin, whatever that may have been, I gave the worse patient *Pyrogen* as in the last case, and *Baptisia* to the less bad one. In three days the patient taking *Pyrogen* was feverless; and the one on *Baptisia?* Her temperature had gone on steadily rising, and was 104° or thereabouts. Why did you not give them both *Pyroge*n said the mother?

I did not enter into the question, but ordered *Pyrogenium* then for the other, and down went the temperature as in the previous case.

This is my experience of *Pyrogenium,* not, indeed, all of it, but the bulk of it.

Now, let those who have more fevers to treat than I have put it to the test, but not in low dilutions, or hypodermically, but in the 6th centesimal by the mouth, as I have done.

But the *Pyrogenium* should not be diluted or preserved with glycerine, but the matrix fluid should be forthwith run up to the 6th centesimal dilution, as is customary in homœopathic pharmaceutics. In other respects it must be prepared as directed by Dr Drysdale in his paper already referred to, and the control experiment on some living creature should be attended to. I will not enlarge upon the subject, but will pass on now to the experience of my friend Dr Shuldham of Putney. The experience of this scholarly and able colleague is singularly opportune and suggestive; it comes to me in the form of a letter, and I leave it to speak for itself, merely saying that it bears out my own idea of the sphere of usefulness of *Pyrogenium* in diphtheria, and is in accordance with Dr Drysdale's theoretical reasoning and suggestion.

The following is Dr Shuldham's letter:—

"ELMSTEAD, CARLTON ROAD, PUTNEY,
"*Feby.* 8, 1888.

"MY DEAR BURNETT,—You ask me for a little news about *Pyrogenium*.

"Here it is.

"First of all I must tell you that the earliest news I had of this medicine was associated with your name. The case was one of typhoid fever, which, according to my patient's account, had been broken up by your timely use of this nosode. The next bit of news in connexion with *Pyrogenium* was that it had been given to a poor consumptive girl by before-mentioned friendly patient, and the girl's temperature had been frequently lowered by the medicine.

"There was no mistake about the temperature, for the girl's mother, an intelligent observer, had used the clinical thermometer.

"I regret to say that there was very little doubt as to the nature of the case, for I attended this very patient in her last sad illness.

"The next bit of news comes of your observations of the medicine.

"It is in this wise,—

"In August 1887 I was attending a little boy for a diphtheritic sore throat, and the boy was not racing his way to recovery. Indeed, matters were at a standstill, when I thought of *Pyrogenium,* and gave it in the sixth dilution—centesimal. But let me first say, by way of parenthesis, that the boy's temperature was $102\frac{1}{2}°$ F. There were patches on both tonsils, the breath was offensive, the tongue thickly furred, and the complexion was muddy. The *Pyrogenium* was given on a Tuesday, and by Wednesday morning there was a marvellous change for the better.

"The temperature had fallen to 99° F., the throat was less inflamed and less covered with membrane. The tongue was cleaner, and the complexion was less muddy.

"The next day matters improved still more, and by Friday I had taken leave of the patient.

"This was not all.

"The little boy's sister was seized with chills, headache, aching in the limbs, and soreness of the throat. The clinical thermometer marked 102½° F. in her case. Suspecting that I had another case of blood-poisoning to deal with, I gave *Pyro.* 6, and by next day all these uncanny symptoms had vanished like a dream.

"I fear, my dear Burnett, I weary you, but at the risk of being thought a dreadful bore. I will add one more experience.

'The mother of my little boy patient nursed her son, and was infected by the same blood poison. False membrane was deposited on both tonsils, the patient had a foul breath, a furred tongue, and a look of weariness and illness that betokened serious trouble. But she only remained in bed two days after having taken the first dose of *Pyro.*, and made a good recovery.

"My first patient, the little boy, was taking the traditional *Belladonna* and *Merc. biniod.* in low dilutions, and was not making progress till *Pyrogenium* came to the rescue.

"I had treated the little patient for a similar attack of sore throat in June, and *Belladonna* and *Merc. iod.* had acted well, so that this masterly inactivity on the part of these medicines made me look for fresh help, which I found, thanks to your previous suggestions, in *Pyro.* 6.

"I gave this medicine in a scarlet fever case just before Christmas on the second day of my attendance, and certainly I had a fall of temperature and a case free from complication, but the results were not so striking as in the diphtheritic cases.

"I shall look forward with great interest to your own experience of this strong power for good.

"With friendly greetings, believe me to be—

"MY DEAR BURNETT,

"Yours very truly,

"E. B. SHULDHAM."

Beyond tendering to Dr Shuldham my thanks for thus giving me the advantage of his experience on this important subject, I will only say that it affords me very great satisfaction to see that every advance in science, wherever it borders on medicine, is sure to redound to the advancement and scientific precision of the law of therapeutics still so foolishly condemned by the majority of mankind.

They have eyes, I suppose, but they see not.

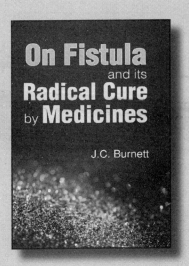

On Fistula and its Radical Cure by Medicines

J. Compton Burnett

- A must have book for every homeopathic practitioner which deals with fistula and abscess, their management and homeopathic medications

- Also includes some case reports for easy grasp of the subject

ISBN: 978-81-319-0785-6 | 112pp | PB

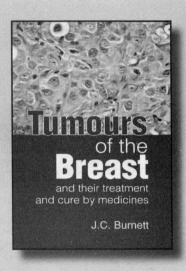

Tumours of the Breast

J. Compton Burnett

- Description of the various kinds of tumors of the breast along with etiology
- Indications of useful homeopathic medicines
- Many clinical cases of different tumors of the breasts along with the treatment given

ISBN: 978-81-319-0768-9 | 128pp | PB

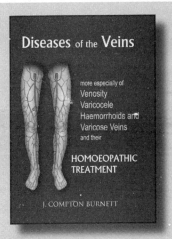

Diseases of the Veins

J. Compton Burnett

- Deals specifically with diseases and disorders of the veins such as varicocele, varicose veins and haemorrhoids (piles)

- The book is divided into two parts - the first being case examples from Dr. Burnett's own practice explaining how he has cured these diseases and the second part being a specific Materia Medica for the treatment of the diseases of the veins

ISBN: 978-81-319-1793-0 | 200pp | PB

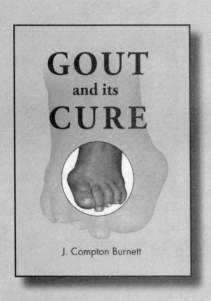

GOUT
and its
CURE

J. Compton Burnett

Gout and its Cure

J. Compton Burnett

- A very useful guide which deals with how to get rid
  of the gouty attack and the deposits and how to deal
  with that which leads to the production of uric acid in
  the body

ISBN: 978-81-319-1790-9 | 184pp | PB

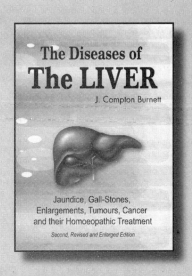

The Diseases of
The LIVER

J. Compton Burnett

Jaundice, Gall-Stones,
Enlargements, Tumours, Cancer
and their Homoeopathic Treatment

Second, Revised and Enlarged Edition

The Diseases of the Liver

J. Compton Burnett

- Precautions and warnings given by great masters of homoeopathy compiled remedy-wise

- Some important tips from clinical records of cures and specific remedies

- Includes and alphabetical repertory at the end of this compilation

ISBN: 978-81-319-1789-3 | 256pp | PB

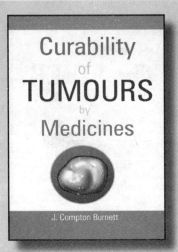

Curability of Tumours by Medicines

J. Compton Burnett

- A comprehensive treatise on the homeopathic treatment of tumours illustrated by detailed case records all throughout

- Beautifully accounts for the causation, clinical characteristics & homeopathic management of tumours with multiple case references

ISBN: 978-81-319-0517-3 | 208pp | PB

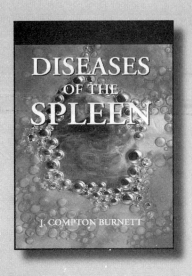

Disease of the Spleen

J. Compton Burnett

- A wonderful compilation of case studies pertaining to various splenic affections and the symptomatologies of the commonly indicated drugs
- Differential diagnosis also mentioned under the cases

ISBN: 978-81-319-0596-8 | 96pp | PB

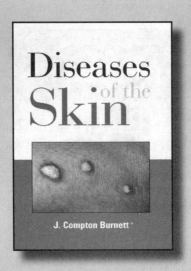

Diseases of the Skin

J. Compton Burnett

- An absorbing account of the great early masters like Boenninghausen and their wonderful contributions to the Homoeopathic Repertory and Materia Medica

- An account of all aspects of prescribing homoeopathic medicines – case taking, case analysis, materia medica, repertorisation, doses and their repetition

ISBN: 978-81-319-0042-0 | 280pp | PB